9 Successful ways to stop Alcoholism

Stop Alcohol and live healthy

Jason J. Williams

1668 Walnut Avenue

Newark, NJ 07102

Table of contents

Chapter nine

Interface with a specialist

The Primary concern

DEDICATION

I want to dedicate this book to almighty God, the creator of heaven and earth, and my family (The Ralph's family), my pastor (Pastor Abel breathe), and my darling wife for always being there for me.

INTRODUCTION

Investigating a couple of changes in your relationship with liquor?

Perhaps you need to:

- ★ Cut how much liquor you drink every week down the middle.

- ★ Restrict yourself to something like two beverages each week.

- ★ Surrender liquor totally, for a set timeframe or forever.

Yet, regardless of your objectives and regardless of the fact that you are so dedicated to improving on your propensities around drinking, keeping away from liquor could demonstrate somewhat more troublesome than you anticipated.

When you settle on the choice to drink all the more carefully or quit drinking completely, you could wind up encountering a few pretty strong desires — especially in spots or circumstances where you'd normally get a brew, present yourself with a glass of wine, or make your effort of decision.

Liquor desires can be exceptionally serious, particularly in early recuperation, makes sense of me been, an authorized clinical social laborer and overseer of clinical activities for advanced recuperation stage Whirlwind.

"The uplifting news is, they just keep going for a brief timeframe. On the off chance that you can divert yourself or endure them, they'll regularly pass."

Underneath, I'll investigate why desires occur and offer a couple of tips to oversee them, from in-the-second procedures to long haul ways of dealing with hardship or stress.

Why desires occur

Desires will not be guaranteed to influence each and every individual who scales back liquor. In any case, they're normal, particularly assuming that you drink consistently or your liquor use falls into the "weighty drinking" classification (hard-core boozing at least 5 days somewhat recently).

Concerning what causes desires? Specialists have recommended at least one or two clarifications.

Changes in cerebrum science

Over the long haul, liquor use starts to influence the synapses, or compound couriers, in your cerebrum.

These progressions can prompt tolerance Trusted Source, or a need to savor more request to feel similar impacts. They can likewise pass on you more delicate to liquor's belongings and raise your gamble of withdrawal side effects.

While not drinking, you could start to see sensations of tension or other close to home pain, areas of strength for alongside for liquor.

Propensity development

Liquor can influence your mind in alternate ways, as well.

Individuals frequently start to utilize liquor routinely on the grounds that drinking prompts good sentiments or works on their temperament:

- A beverage after a horrendous battle with your accomplice could assist you with feeling more quiet.

- A beverage following a difficult day at work could assist you with unwinding.

- A beverage at a party could assist you with conversing with individuals all the more without any problem.

The charming happiness you experience while drinking

turns into a prize, one that supports your longing to savor specific circumstances. You could ultimately begin hankering that award in new circumstances.

CHAPTER 1

Triggers

Desires frequently occur as a programmed reaction to a trigger, which could be a memory of something related with liquor or an inclination like pressure.

The vast majority who experience desires notice a blend of inside and outer triggers.

Inside triggers typically include recollections, contemplations, feelings, or actual impressions that brief the desire to drink.

For instance:

- ★ Misery
- ★ Uneasiness or stress
- ★ Outrage or bothering
- Actual agony or uneasiness

Outside triggers allude to the ecological prompts you connect to liquor, including places, times, individuals, and circumstances.

For instance:

- ★ Visiting an eatery or bar where you normally drink
- ★ Going to a party

★ The finish of your typical working day

★ Contending with a parent

Things to attempt at the time

While a desire for liquor strikes, a decent initial step includes recognizing the hankering. I proceeded to make sense of that while the desire may be extraordinary, it will decrease and pass in almost no time.

"An ordinary desire could keep going for 3 to 5 minutes," notes Christina Hanks, senior recuperation mentor and care group supervisor at Whirlwind.

Advising yourself that the hankering will ease all alone can make it simpler to overcome those minutes without drinking. These systems can help, as well.

CHAPTER 2

Divert yourself

A positive interruption can assist with involving your contemplations and energy, giving you something to zero in on other than the desire to drink.

Hanks suggests making a rundown of interruptions you can go to while a hankering hits and keeping that rundown some place you can get to it rapidly — on your telephone, the cooler, or in a diary, for instance.

A couple of exercises to consider:

- Put on some music and dance.

- Get a book and perused a part.

- Take a stroll, without anyone else or with a companion or pet.

- Watch something interesting.

- Make a bite or cup of tea.

- Clear out a cabinet.

- Attempt some careful shading.

- Invest some energy on your #1 side interest.

Other supportive interruptions could incorporate contemplation, calling a clearheaded pal, or washing up, Hank recommends.

CHAPTER 3

Contact a companion

Checking in with someone else in your life who's attempting to quit drinking can surely assist you with braving a hankering with somebody who comprehends.

However, in any event, when you don't know any other person attempting to roll out a comparative improvement, companions and friends and family can in any case offer basic encouragement.

Indeed, even 10 minutes making up for lost time with late news and sharing stories from your regular routine can offer a sufficient interruption that the desire passes, nearly in a flash.

CHAPTER 4

Remain present

You could see distressing or tense circumstances will generally fuel desires as a rule.

Assuming that is an ideal case for you, care activities can assist you with mooring your mindfulness right now and mitigate yourself until the desire passes.

A couple of thoughts to attempt:

- Profound breathing or unwinding works out.

- Establishing methods

- Actual work, including yoga or stretches.

- Changing your current circumstance.

CHAPTER 5

Embrace interest.

Instead of preparing yourself to confront a hankering with a feeling of limitation, Hanks suggests moving toward the desire with interest.

You could tell yourself, for instance, "I can't help thinking about how traveling through this desire without drinking would feel."

It could likewise assist with tending to your mind straightforwardly (regardless of whether you feel somewhat hesitant). Hanks recommends something as per, "I hear you need a beverage, yet we're having a go at a novel, new thing. We should perceive how it feels."

Long haul techniques

Adapting tips can totally offer momentary arrangements while you're attempting to scale back liquor. All things considered, forever changing your relationship with liquor might require a more inside and out approach.

CHAPTER 6

Figure out your triggers

Carving out opportunity to investigate the particular individuals, spots, and circumstances that prompt your inclination to drink can have a major effect.

"At the point when we experience things that help us to remember a drinking episode, we can encounter powerful desires.

I noticed that it can assist with keeping away from your triggers however much as could reasonably be expected in early recuperation, since triggers are in many cases most extreme when you first quit drinking.

Staying away from triggers could mean:

★ Moving your wine rack to the storm cellar or giving it to a companion.

★ Picking cafes that don't serve liquor.

★ Pending time with companions now and again you don't connect with drinking switching around your drive to try not to pass your #1 bar.

★ Rehearsing great taking care of oneself to address

needs for rest, food, water, and friendship.

Obviously, tending to your triggers at the source can likewise go far toward assisting you with rolling out enduring improvements.

Perhaps you experience your most grounded desires when you feel restless or pushed or wind up confronting struggle with somebody you care about.

Figuring out how to manage troublesome feelings and handle these difficulties in additional useful ways can work on your connections and generally prosperity, also assist with decreasing the desire to drink.

CHAPTER 7

Construct your own customized tool compartment

Similarly as various things can set off liquor desires from one individual to another, various procedures can assist you with overseeing them.

At the end of the day, what works for a companion will not necessarily work for you. That is the reason constructing your own recuperation tool compartment can have an effect in your capacity to climate the most powerful desires.

You could try and have two distinct tool compartments:

- A real actual box or pack that incorporates things like a consoling book, a most loved nibble, a cherished belonging, or a diary

- An "imperceptible" toolbox of things you can't see or contact, similar to your #1 care or breathing activities, expressions of self-empathy, and certifying mantras

"Long haul, we're fabricating a wellbeing net around ourselves," Hanks says.

"You are at the focal point of your recuperation, and it can assist with outlining it as a demonstration of inventiveness. You're painting your own recuperation process, and stroke by stroke, you're learning better ways of adapting."

CHAPTER 8

End the propensity circle

Assuming that you've at any point attempted to get out from under any propensity, you most likely know it's frequently easy to talk about, not so easy to do.

Understanding the three particular parts of your propensity circle can assist you with concocting more unambiguous systems to conquer desires when they spring up.

- To begin with, there's the prompt, or trigger — the main twinge of nervousness before a date, or a disturbing email from your chief.

- Then there's the everyday practice — having a glass or two of wine with your flat mate when you both return home from work, or requesting a beverage with supper.

- Lastly, the prize that supports the propensity — a wonderful buzz, a superior state of mind, or a drop in your feelings of anxiety.

When you distinguish the signs, schedules, and rewards that keep your propensity circle on a recurrent cycle, you can explore different avenues regarding new schedules that yield considerably additional satisfying prizes.

Find out about making the propensity circle work for you.

CHAPTER 9

Interface with a specialist

Treatment with a prepared emotional wellness proficient — especially one who spends significant time in substance use and recuperation — can be one more extraordinary method for investigating long haul changes in liquor use.

A specialist can offer help with:

- Unloading explicit necessities you use liquor to help satisfy.

- Investigating substitute strategies for taking care of pressure.

- Distinguishing any emotional wellness side effects or rest concerns you attempt to deal with liquor.

Advisors can likewise show new care systems and adapting procedures, alongside mental conduct strategies you can use to challenge and reexamine negative contemplations or self-convictions connected to liquor desires.

How drug can help

Liquor desires can be challenging to oversee alone, and there's no disgrace in requiring some additional help.

Prescription is one extra choice for dealing with serious

and industrious desires:

- ★ Naltrexone (Vivitrol, Revia) works by restricting to your endorphin receptors and obstructing liquor's belongings. It can assist with diminishing desires, decrease the sum you drink, and make it simpler to keep up with collectedness once you quit drinking.

- ★ Acamprosate (Campral) likewise diminishes desires, however some exploration recommends it very well might be somewhat more powerful for proceeding with balance after you've previously quit drinking. This drug seems to assist with reestablishing liquor related uneven characters in cerebrum science and straightforwardness withdrawal side effects.

- ★ Disulfram (Antabuse) doesn't straightforwardly forestall desires. Rather, it can cause you to feel less like drinking since it makes it challenging for your body to process liquor. On the off chance that you drink while taking this medicine, you'll encounter various upsetting and undesirable impacts, including sickness and spewing, migraine, dampness, from there, the sky is the limit. It's not recommended as frequently as it used to be, yet it's as yet a choice.

Keen on attempting drug for liquor desires? A specialist or therapist can offer more data and assist you with investigating conceivable treatment plans.

Certain antidepressants likewise show promiseTrusted Hotspot for decreasing drinking when you live with despondency. Your consideration group could suggest this methodology in the event that you experience side effects of uneasiness and despondency alongside desires.

The primary concern

Liquor desires are normal, particularly when you first attempt to change your drinking propensities. It could require an investment and work to find a methodology that assists you with exploring them successfully, yet you really do have a lot of choices for help.

Treatment, prescription, and recuperation projects can all have benefit for decreasing and forestalling desires. Consolidating drug with treatment and different intercessions can demonstrate much more supportive than medicine alone.

By the day's end, simply recollect you don't need to run the course alone — interfacing with a specialist or joining a recuperation program can have a significant effect.